Sunny Cabana Publishing, L.L.C.

The Vivacious Vegan Desserts

Just because you choose a vegan diet doesn't mean you have to deprive yourself of dessert! You have choices!

By Kathy Tennefoss

The Vivacious Vegan Desserts
Sunny Cabana Publishing, L.L.C.
Fort Lauderdale, FL

www.sunnycabanapublishing.com
facebook.com/sunnycabanapublishing

Authored by Kathy Tennefoss

All Rights Reserved © 2011 by Kathy Tennefoss
No part of this book may be reproduced or transmitted in any form by any means, graphic, electronic, or mechanical, including photocopying, recording, taping, or by any information storage or retrieval system, without permission in writing from the publisher.
Published by Kathleen Tennefoss
Printed in the United States of America
Author: Kathy Tennefoss
Photography Kathy Tennefoss
Illustrator Rin Kurhana
13-digit ISBN: 9781936874187
10-digit ISBN: 1936874180
First Printing

This book is dedicated to everyone who wants to make a difference in the world by eating a vegan diet, either full or part time. Any type of commitment you make to improve the planet and your health is life changing for yourself and others. Don't wait until your health fails start now! Your friends and family will thank you!

Cover Design Kathy Tennefoss

Photos Kathy Tennefoss

Cover Illustrations by Rin Kurohana

First edition, 2011

Acknowledgements:

Thanks to everyone who encouraged, inspired, and gave me excellent input and feedback, and especially to my wonderful husband who had to endear my countless trial dessert runs! Without everyone's input I would not have finished this book. I am extremely grateful to everyone and I hope that this book helps others to eat healthy and to be active in their daily life!

If you have any suggestions, comments, or corrections please send me an email to sunnycabanapublishing@gmail.com.

Like us on facebook.com/sunnycabanapublishing!

www.SunnyCabanaPublishing.com

SunnyCabanaPublishing@gmail.com or

TheVivaciousVegan@gmail.com

Contents

Intro Page 7

Some Concerns for a Vegan Diet Page 11

Are You Getting the Correct Amount of Nutrients? Page 13

What's The Deal with Sugar? Page 15

What's The Deal with Flour? Page 19

Stocking the Kitchen Page 21

Cakes, Bread, & Muffins Page 25

Cookies & Candies Page 49

Pies & Puddings Page 71

Frozen Treats Page 85

Sweet Drinks Page 105

Some Helpful Vegan Websites Page 115

Some Helpful Phone Apps Page 117

Vegan Schools and Cooking Classes Page 119

Index Page 125

Intro

I know what you are thinking. Vegan desserts isn't that an oxymoron? Well not really! Vegans you can have your cake and eat it too! It seems that the more I talk to people the one thing that they can't seem to modify is desserts. Most say if I had better vegan dessert choices I would be 100% vegan. The world is changing ever so quickly and there are so many new products that are available for vegans like soy cream cheese or tofu cream cheese, soy whip, Ricemallow, nut and grain milks, soy butter (Earth Balance), soy yogurt, soy ice cream, and many other new and tasty ingredients that are worthy of trying!

You don't have to eat vegan everyday but it is a good way to eat if you want to lose or maintain your weight, eat heart healthy, help the environment, and save the lives of animals!

I have been interested in the health industry for over 20 years and feel that eating a healthy diet, exercising, and having fun are the key components to living a long life!

Don't be too hard on yourself if you slip on your diet; remember you are only human you have to allow for change and improvement. Maybe it's just taking eggs out of your diet this month and then next month its cheese, whatever works for you to improve your life and your health. Everyone is different and responds differently to diets so just because your friend or family member is able to eat a certain way does not mean that you will or that your body will respond in the same way. Keep an open mind and an open heart when you are changing anything in your life! This may make all the difference in the world! But really the most important thing is to have fun trying new recipes and sharing them with your friends and family!

Like us on Facebook:

facebook.com/sunnycabanapublishing

www.SunnyCabanaPublishing.com

Email SunnyCabanapublishing@gmail.com or TheVivaciousVegan@gmail.com

Some Concerns for a Vegan Diet

Are you getting enough B-12?

One thing that a person should take into account if they are on a vegan diet is that they should make sure they are getting enough B-12 in their diet. **<u>B-12 can only be found naturally in animal products!</u>** This is extremely important due to the fact that it sometimes takes 1-5 years before you even notice that you are not getting enough B-12. Here are some signs: anemia, nervous system damage, depression, loss of energy, tingling, numbness, poor memory, confusion, & personality changes. You may not even know that some of these signs are from the inadequate amounts of B-12, but it is always a good idea to get your blood work done to make sure you are in a healthy state!

One thing that can throw off your blood work if you already are a vegan or raw foodie is if you consume algae or spirulina it can change your blood work to give you a false reading because algae contains b-12 analogues but not the correct ones that are needed for b-12 deficiency. So make sure you tell your doctor if you are taking these supplements before your test.

Some also say that if you eat nori, tempeh, or barley grass you will get enough B-12 to sustain your body. I think that it is best to just make sure you are getting the correct amount by either taking a B-12 supplement or by eating foods or plant milks that are fortified with B-12 to make sure you are getting the required amount of 2-3 mcgs a day of B-12 and if you are pregnant make sure it's closer to the 3 mcgs a day. Make sure you do check with your doctor to make sure these are the correct doses for your body type or if you have any other ailments that may interfere with this dosage.

Are you getting the correct amount of nutrients?

Everything should be eaten with balance! Make sure you have the right amount of protein ratio to carbohydrates and eat lots of veggies and fruits! If you are not eating dairy, meat, fish, and eggs you will be getting your protein from nuts, tofu, soy products, quinoa, seeds, & beans. Your carbohydrates should be brown rice, millet, bulgur, whole wheat or other plant based pastas. And the fruits and veggies are self explanatory! Mix it up! Just eat as many veggies as you can a day. If you don't like to eat veggies that much try hiding them in smoothies or soups (especially for little ones)! Don't think you have to just sit down and eat a whole pile of kale to get your nutrition. When you eat veggies and fruits you will feel full; plus veggies have a lot fewer calories than packaged food!

Some may say that you can't get enough calcium if you don't eat dairy products. You can get calcium from dark green leafy vegetables, fortified orange juices or plant based milks, or fortified tofu. There is more calcium in ¾ cup of collard greens than in a full cup of regular milk. So vegans don't be afraid that you are not getting enough calcium just eat your dark leafy greens! I think that the best way to do this is by eating them in your smoothies! You should be getting anywhere from 1000-12000 mg a day depending on your age and sex.

Unsulfured black strap molasses has almost 400 mg for only 2 tablespoons and 1 cup of cooked collard greens has 350 mgs of calcium and 1 cup of tofu or tempeh has around 200 mgs also so you can see that it wouldn't be too hard to get your daily intake of calcium from a vegan diet!

What's The Deal with Sugar?

Most Americans consume 2-3 pounds of refined sugar a week. It seems so crazy to me that people are not aware of the hidden refined sugars in foods; like in sauces, packaged foods, dressings, etc. Refined sugars raise insulin levels in the blood making a person more prone to diabetes. Refined sugar also promotes the storage of fat in the body, which translates into weight gain. Refined sugar can also raise triglycerides in your cholesterol. Refined sugar can also cause hyperactivity, anxiety, depression, difficulty concentrating, and many other not so good things for your body. This is not a good thing. Refined sugar also has no nutritional value; no minerals or vitamins! It actually takes nutrients away from your body by even processing it! There are better natural substitutes out there that have a higher nutritional value and taste great too. But as with anything you still have to watch how much you intake, even if it is natural.

As far as sweeteners go one of my favorite sweeteners to use is Agave (cactus) Nectar. I use it in smoothies and in my green tea but there are many other ways to sweeten your food naturally.

You can use date sugar (or if you don't have date sugar you may use just pitted dates) which, is made of ground up dried dates and by using date sugar you have added fiber to your recipe. What a bonus! You can also use other dried fruits that are ground up in a food processor. You will just have to experiment to see what you like best. I have used this on occasion. If I have dates on hand I will use one or two in my morning green smoothies! They give you an extra boost of energy for working out!

Another one of my favorites is maple syrup because it mixes well in liquids and has tons of minerals and a great flavor. Plus it's really good on vegan pancakes!

Turbinado sugar is another good choice that is made from partially refined raw sugar, which can be better if you want a smoother finish in a dessert or smoothie.

Another type of sweetener that can be used in vegan dishes is called barley malt syrup. Barley malt syrup is very thick and tastes a lot like molasses. Barley malt syrup is made from whole grain barley by sprouting it which creates enzymes that are good for your body!

Another great tasting sweetener is organic brown rice syrup. Brown rice syrup can be substituted for maple syrup, honey, corn syrup, sugar, or molasses. Use ¼ cup of rice syrup for one cup of sugar and then use ¼ cup less of another liquid in the recipe.

So all in all you won't really miss refined sugar if you just follow the above choices for your recipes. Plus you are adding more minerals, fiber, enzymes, and amino acids to your diet. So life can be sweeter for you!

Using refined sugars are not beneficial to the body because it imbalances the body gives you an energy crash. Companies have been trying to manufacture sweeteners like saccharine and aspartame, which have reports of being taken off the market for being toxic or causing cancer, either way it doesn't sound that great when there are tons of natural alternatives out there in the supermarket. You will end up spending a bit more for these natural sugar substitutes but isn't your health worth it!

What's The Deal with Flour?

There are so many different flours out there that you can use for your recipes but one that is not as great for your health is bleached white flour. Bleached white flour is missing the germ and the bran from the grain, which is the nutritious part of the grain. They are loaded with fiber which as you should know fiber is good for your body! You should eat anywhere from 30-40 grams of fiber a day in order to help ward off such diseases as high cholesterol, obesity, high blood sugar, colon cancer (or any other type of cancer) and heart disease. Deciding on a high fiber diet is going to cause some changes simply because your body doesn't understand a sudden change. You could experience headaches, constipation, nausea, or diarrhea when first starting to eat healthy foods. If you get your fiber from raw foods, there is a much less chance of adverse effects, but no guarantees.

Amaranth flour can be used for baking and it is high in protein, fiber, and vitamins. Amaranth has a nutty flavor so it does work well for baking.

Buckwheat flour is also high in fiber and protein but it has a heavier taste and can be used for things like pancakes.

Brown rice flour can be used also but it should be mixed with other flours because it tends to crumble a bit more.

Nut flours like almond meal are another great source of flour. Almond meal gives the recipe a great flavor plus it also gives it higher protein content. Almond meal can also be used as a non dairy powder replacement for many recipes.

Sprouted flour is one of the best flours that you can use for your health. Sprouted flours such as rye, spelt, wheat, have higher fiber content, are easier to digest, have increased vitamin C, B, and enzymes.

Freshly ground grain flour will last 3-4 months on the shelf. In the refrigerator it will last 6-8 months and in the freezer it will last around 14 months. When in doubt throw it out!

Stocking the Kitchen

Here are some things that you may need in order to succeed with vegan desserts!

- Baking Sheets
- Baking Pans
- Pie Pan (either glass of metal; I prefer glass)
- Muffin Tins & Liners
- Micro plane & Grater
- Spatulas of all kinds (You can never have too many!)
- Peeler
- Whisk
- Sifter
- Rolling Pin
- Colander
- Parchment Paper
- Aluminum Foil
- Plastic Wrap
- Wax Paper
- Toothpicks
- Blender

- Vitamixer (This is my equipment of choice)
- Food Processor
- Ice Cream Maker
- Juicer
- Measuring Cups & Spoons
- Mixing Bowls

Always try to keep as many fresh fruits, veggies, spices, frozen fruits, nuts, seeds, nut butters, apple sauce, vinegar, Arrowroot, natural flavored extracts, soy, nut, and grain milks, vegan margarine (my favorite is Earth Balance), soy cream cheese, soy yogurt, soy ice cream, semi-chocolate chips or cocoa powder, vegan marshmallows, agave nectar, maple syrup, dates, coconut, oats, wheat germ, spelt flour, whole wheat pastry flour, chestnut flour, garbanzo flour, almond meal, Ener-G egg replacer powder, brown rice syrup, cocoa nibs (I love these things), graham cracker crumbs or pie shells, tofu, and organic turbinado sugar. Really anything that you can make vegan goodies out of!

Some egg substitutes that you can use in these recipes and in your own would be 3 tablespoons of applesauce, ½ smashed banana, or 1 tablespoon of flaxseeds ground (I like using the golden ones because the color is better with most baked goods) with 2 tablespoons of water. There is also the Ener-G egg replacer which works really well!

Cakes, Breads, & Muffins

Chocolate Pineapple Coffee Cake

Banana Nut Bread

Plantain Coconut Cake

Vanilla Orange Cake

Nutty Carrot Cake

Pecan Blueberry Muffins

Raspberry White Chocolate Chip Muffins

Cup Cakes

Fluffy Frosting

Jalapeno Cornbread

Chocolate Pineapple Coffee Cake

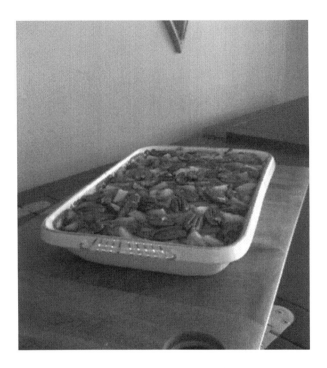

Make sure that you do all of these steps before putting into the oven. The coffee cake is cooked with the sauce and topping! This is one of my favorites!

Preheat the oven to 350 degrees

Cake: Dry Ingredients

2 ¼ Cups organic unbleached white flour

1 ½ teaspoon baking soda

1 ½ non- aluminum baking powder

½ teaspoon of salt

1 cup semi sweet chocolate chips

Wet Ingredients:

1 ½ Cup hemp vanilla milk

4 ½ Tablespoons of maple syrup

¾ teaspoon of pure vanilla extract

3 Tablespoons of organic safflower oil

1 ½ Tablespoons of organic apple cider

Shift the dry ingredients and then mix the liquid ingredients in a separate bowl. Now blend the mixture and put into an oiled 9 x 10 pan.

Next make the topping:

1 ½ cup pineapple

1 cup whole pecans

Take these ingredients and place them on the top of the batter.

Now add the sauce:

½ Cup organic barley malt syrup

½ Cup organic maple syrup

3 Tablespoons of ground cinnamon

½ Cup organic safflower oil

Mix the above sauce ingredients and pour on the batter and bake at 350 degrees for 45 minutes or till golden brown.

Let this coffee cake cool and serve at your next vegan brunch and better yet don't tell anyone that its vegan! Yum!

Another alternative is to not put the pineapple on top and use 1 ½ cups of chocolate chips! It will be good either way!

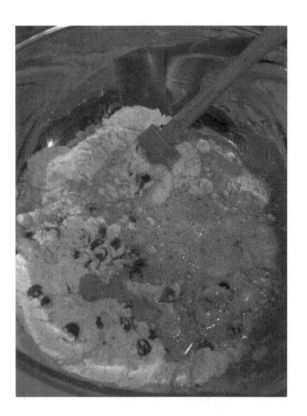

Banana Nut Bread

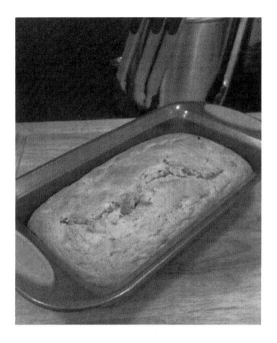

3 Cups Whole Wheat Flour

1Tablespoon of cinnamon

3 Teaspoons of aluminum free baking powder

1 Teaspoon of baking power

½ Pecans chopped

1 Cup Maple Syrup

3 Ripe bananas

½ Applesauce

¼ Cup apple juice

Preheat oven to 350 degrees. Mix dry ingredients first. Then mash the bananas up in another bowl and add the rest of the ingredients. Next fold the batter into the dry mixture. Mix well and then pour into a greased loaf pan and bake for 45-50 minutes or until golden brown. It may take a few extra minutes so don't worry if you have to end up cooking it for one full hour. Just keep an eye on it!

Plantain Coconut Cake

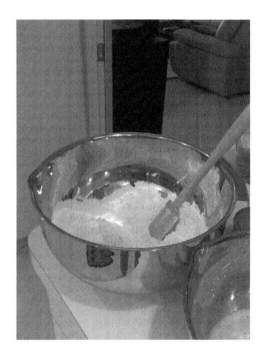

1½ Cup whole wheat flour

1 Teaspoon non aluminum baking powder

½ Non sulfured shredded coconut

2 Very ripe plantains

¼ Cup brown sugar

1/3 Cup raw sugar

1 Teaspoon vanilla

Topping:

1 Tablespoon of safflower oil

½ Cup non sulfured shredded coconut

1/3 Cup chopped almonds

3 Tablespoons of almond milk

Heat oven to 350 degrees. Mix flour, baking powder and coconut. Mash plantains, sugars, and vanilla. Mix together both ingredients until smooth. Place the batter into a greased cake pan. Bake for 30 minutes. Cool. Then take the topping ingredients and mix together and pour on cake and broil for a few minutes until golden brown. Serve!

Vanilla Orange Cake

2 ½ Cups all purpose flour

2 Teaspoons of non aluminum baking powder

½ Teaspoon baking soda

2 Cups powdered sugar

½ Earth Balance

1 ¾ Cups almond milk

2 Tablespoons orange juice (1/2 orange)

1 Orange peel grated

1 Tablespoon vanilla extract

1 Teaspoon white vinegar

Preheat oven to 350 degrees. Grease and flour two round cake pans. Combine flour, baking powder, and baking soda in a bowl. Next cream together Earth Balance and the powdered sugar. Add the almond milk, orange juice, orange peel, vinegar, and vanilla. Mix this mixture with the flour until smooth. Pour into the baking pans and bake for 20-25 minutes or until golden brown or a tooth pick comes out clean. Dust with a bit of powdered sugar or frost with your favorite vegan icing.

Nutty Carrot Cake

2 ¼ Cup all purpose flour

1 Tablespoon non aluminum baking powder

1 Teaspoon baking powder

1 Teaspoon salt

1 Cup raw sugar

1 Cup safflower oil

¾ Cup maple syrup

1/3 Cup hazelnut milk

3 Tablespoons of hemp seeds

4 Tablespoons applesauce

1 Tablespoon cinnamon

1 teaspoon vanilla extract

2 Cups shredded carrots

½ Cup chopped and pitted dates

½ Cup raisins

½ Cup walnuts

1 orange grated

Icing:

1 ½ Cup powdered sugar

1 Cup soy cream cheese

½ Cup Earth Balance

1 Teaspoon vanilla

Preheat oven to 350 degrees. Grease a 9 by 13 inch baking dish. Add all the dry ingredients EXCEPT sugar. In another bowl mix the sugar, oil, maple sugar, hazelnut milk, and applesauce. Add the rest of the ingredients to the sugar mixture and then fold into the dry ingredients. Pour into the baking dish and bake for 40-45 minutes. Cool fully and then make the frosting and serve immediately!

Pecan Blueberry Muffins

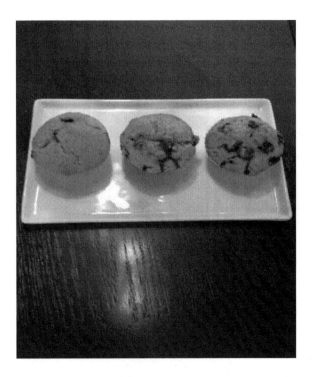

These are one of my favorites!

¼ Cup Earth Balance

½ Plus 1/8 Cup of organic applesauce

½ Teaspoon salt

1 Cup Sugar

2 Cups all purpose organic flour

1 Tablespoon non aluminum baking powder

1 Teaspoon vanilla

¾ Cup of hazelnut milk

2 Cup frozen blueberries

½ Cup chopped pecans

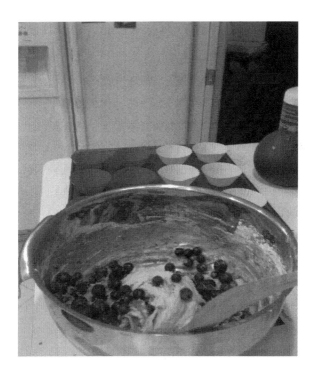

Preheat the oven to 350 degrees. Next take the sugar and Earth Balance and mix together.

Start to add the applesauce, vanilla, and hazelnut milk. Take the flour, baking powder and salt and mix in another bowl. Now blend the ingredients together. The dough will be sticky and hard to mix. Add the blueberries and pecans and fill the muffin tins or I use the silicon ones. Really it's your choice. Bake at 350 degrees for around 40 minutes or until golden brown. Cool and serve! This recipe makes 12. Make sure you fill the muffin tins full because they will not raise as much as a regular muffin recipe.

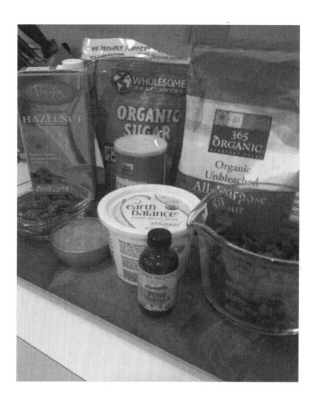

Raspberry & White Chocolate Chip Muffins

Cup Earth Balance

½ Plus 1/8 Cup of organic applesauce

½ Teaspoon salt

1 Cup Sugar

2 Cups all purpose organic flour

1 Tablespoon non aluminum baking powder

1 Teaspoon vanilla

¾ Cup of hazelnut milk

2 Cup frozen Raspberries

1 Cup Vegan White Chocolate Chips (you can order them online at www.veganstore.com or many other vegan stores online)

Preheat the oven to 350 degrees. Next take the sugar and Earth Balance and mix together. Start to add the applesauce, vanilla, and hazelnut milk. Take the flour, baking powder and salt and mix in another bowl. Now blend the ingredients together. The dough will be sticky and hard to mix. Add the raspberries and vegan white chocolate chips and fill a muffin tin or I use the silicon ones. Really it's your choice. Bake at 350 degrees for around 40 minutes or until golden brown. Cool and serve! They make about 12. Make sure to fill the muffin tins almost to the top. It will seem like too much but they do not raise as much as a regular muffin.

Cup Cakes

2 Cups all purpose flour

1 Cup sugar

2 Teaspoons of non aluminum baking powder

½ Teaspoon of baking soda

½ Teaspoon of salt

½ Cup safflower oil

1 Teaspoon of vanilla

1 Tablespoon apple cider vinegar

1 ½ Almond milk

Heat oven to 350 degrees. Use either silicon or tin muffin holders. I prefer silicon but it's up to you. If you do use a tin muffin pan make sure to grease and flour the bottom of the pan. Add the apple cider to the almond milk and let sit for a few minutes. While that is sitting you can mix the dry ingredients together and then in another bowl mix in the liquid ingredients. Now fold the liquid ingredients into the dry ingredients. Next pour the mixture into the muffin tins 9t should make 12-15 cupcakes. Bake for 15-20 minutes. Make sure they don't get too brown. Take them out when done and cool on a cooling rack.

You can either frost them or not.

Vegan Frosting

¾ Cup Earth Balance

¼ Cup vanilla soy creamer

1 ½ Teaspoon vanilla extract

3 ½ Cups of powdered sugar

Mix all ingredients until smooth and fluffy. Once you have your cupcakes cooled you can place the frosting in a large Ziploc bag to use as a piping bag to frost your cupcakes.

*Another fun thing to do is to add chopped up vegan chocolate cookie, vegan candy, or chopped peppermint!

Jalapeno Cornbread

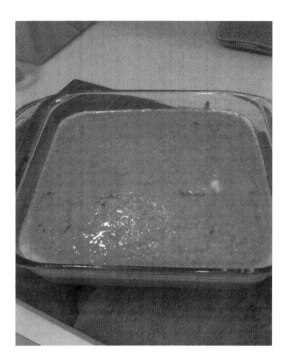

1 ½ Cups organic yellow cornmeal (preferably fine ground but you can use medium for a denser bread or what I do is use ½ medium and ½ fine ground cornmeal)

1 ¼ Cup organic unbleached flour

1 Teaspoon salt

2 Teaspoons of non aluminum baking powder

1 Tablespoon apple cider vinegar

½ Cup maple syrup

¼ Cup Safflower oil

1 ½ Cups almond milk

1-2 Finely chopped Jalapenos (depending on how hot you like it)

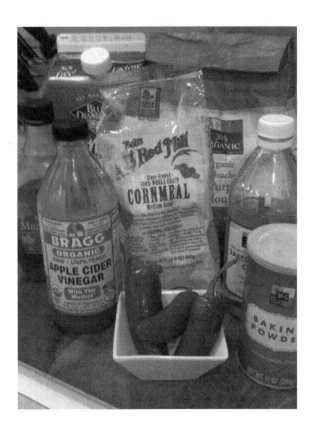

Topping:

Mix equal parts agave nectar with Earth Balance and mix until fluffy. Use it to put on top of the bread when done or just use in on each slice.

Heat oven to 350 degrees. Oil and cornmeal the bottom of an 8 x 8 pan. Combine dry ingredients in a bowl and then combine the liquid ingredients in another bowl and then mix together. Then add the jalapenos. Bake for 35-40 minutes or until a fork comes out clean.

Cookies & Candies

Lemony Bars

Chocolate Fudge

Chocolate Brownies

Date & Raisin Trail Droppings

Chewy Oatmeal Cookies

Almond & Peanut Brittle

Peanut Butter Cookies

Almond Cookies

Everything Bars

Lemony Bars

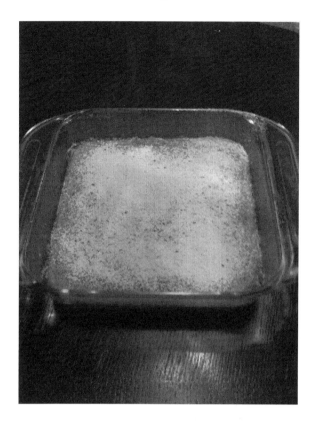

Crust:

½ Cup Earth Balance

¼ Cup powdered sugar

1 Cup all purpose flour

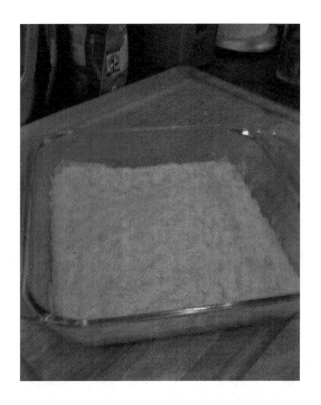

Filling:

½ Cup Silken tofu

1 Cup sugar

Zest from 3 lemons

½ Cup lemon juice

2 Tablespoons of flour

4 Tablespoons arrowroot

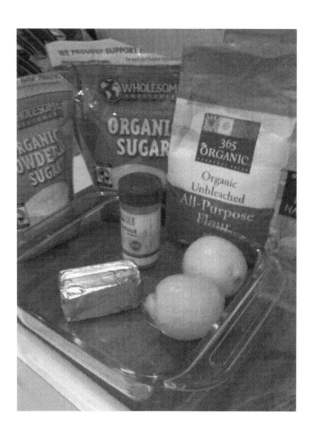

Preheat oven to 350 degrees. Use an 8x8 glass baking pan. Make sure to grease it and lightly flour the bottom of the pan. Cream together the Earth Balance and powdered sugar and then add the flour. Press this mixture into the pan and bake for 20 minutes. Now mix the filling. Blend the rest of the ingredients until smooth and creamy and pour into the crust shell and bake again for 30-35 minutes. Cool and then dust with powdered sugar and serve! Make sure to refrigerate the bars to keep them fresh.

Chocolate Fudge

1 Jar of rice mellow fluff

1 ½ Cup powdered sugar

2/3 Cup of hazelnut milk

¼ Cup Earth Balance

½ Teaspoon of salt

3 ½ Cups of semi sweet chocolate chips

1 Teaspoon of vanilla

1 Cup chopped walnuts

First oil a 9x10 pan. Next take the rice mellow fluff, salt, Earth Balance, hazelnut milk, and powdered sugar and heat on low heat until smooth. Next take the chocolate chips and vanilla and mix them into the heated mixture. Only leave this on the stove for a couple of minutes. Now pour into the pan and top with the walnuts. Refrigerate for 3 hours or freeze if you like to have it frozen. It tastes great either way.

Chocolaty Brownies

2 Cups sugar

2 Cups all purpose flour

¾ Cup of cocoa powder

1 Teaspoon of non aluminum powder

1 Teaspoon salt

1 Cup almond milk

1 Cup Safflower oil

1 Teaspoon of vanilla extract

½ Cup peanut butter chips

½ Semi sweet chocolate chips

Preheat oven to 350 degrees. Mix dry ingredients in a bowl first and then add everything except the chips. Blend until smooth and then pour into a greased 9 x 13 pan and top with the chips. Bake for 25-30 minutes. Let cool and then serve.

Date & Raisin Oatmeal Trail Droppings

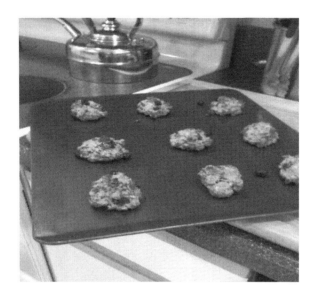

These are hearty! I would take these on a camping trip.

Dry Ingredients:

2 Cups organic oats

¾ Cup organic whole wheat pastry flour

¾ Cup organic unbleached white flour

2 teaspoons of non aluminum baking powder

1 teaspoon of cinnamon

½ teaspoon of sea salt

½ Cup seedless raisins

½ Cup (4 dates) pitted and chopped dates

1 Cup chopped walnuts

Wet Ingredients:

½ Cup organic safflower oil

1 Cup organic apple juice

¼ Cup organic maple syrup

2 Tablespoons of organic barley malt syrup

1 Teaspoon of pure vanilla extract

Preheat oven to 400 degrees. Mix dry ingredients in a separate bowl and then mix wet ingredients and then combine together. The mixture may be a bit dry if it is just add a bit more of the apple juice to get the right consistency.

Oil baking sheets. Spoon cookies onto the sheet with about 2 inches between them and bake for 15-18 minutes. Cool and enjoy!

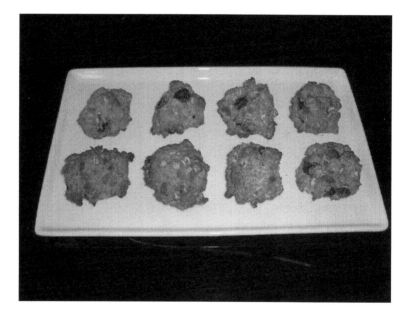

Chewy Oatmeal, Raisin, & Pecan Cookies

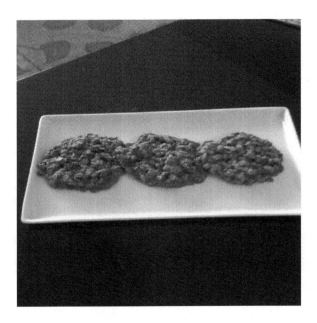

These are another one of my favorites! I grew up in Akron, Ohio and I used to go to Quaker Square for oatmeal cookies all of the time. These are the closest that I could come to them and they are vegan! Yum.

Ingredients:

¾ Cup Earth Balance

1/3 Cup organic sugar

¾ Cup brown sugar

½ Cup Hazelnut Milk (or whatever vegan milk you have; I just like the taste of the hazelnut milk better)

1 teaspoon of vanilla

1 Cup organic flour

½ teaspoon of baking soda

1 teaspoon of cinnamon

3 Cups organic oats or oat flakes

1 Cup raisins

½ Cup chopped pecans

First earth balance and the sugars and mixed well and then add the hazelnut milk and vanilla. Now take the dry ingredients and mix well and then combine with the wet ingredients. Now spoon the cookies onto an ungreased cookie sheet and bake at 350 degrees for around 12 minutes. They will be large and a little flat but they are really chewy and taste great!

*Tip: Do not leave too long on the baking sheet to cool otherwise the will stick and it will be hard to lift them. Wait about a minute or two and just be very careful when you lift them off the sheet! They are a bit fragile.

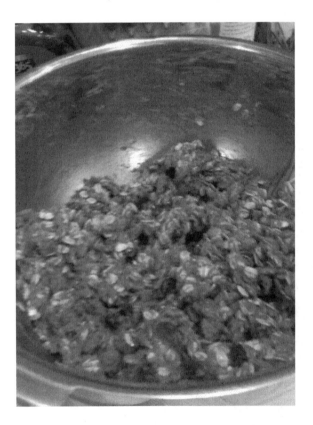

Almond & Peanut Brittle

1 ½ Cup dry roasted peanuts

1 ½ Cup Dry Roasted Almonds

1 Cup sugar

1 Cup organic brown rice syrup

1 Teaspoon baking soda

1 Teaspoon Earth Balance

Grease a large baking pan. Combine sugar and brown rice syrup together in a sauce pan and heat to a boiling temperature. Make sure that you are stirring constantly! Continue boiling until the temp is 300 degrees. When the sugars begin to turn brown add the nut. Make sure they are all coated. Turn off the heat and add the Earth Balance and baking soda. Now pour onto the greased baking pan. When it is cool enough to touch try to stretch the mixture out flat on the baking sheet. Cool and then break into small pieces. Another alternative is to drizzle melted semi chocolate chips on top and then break it up into pieces! Either way it's good.

Peanut Butter Cookies

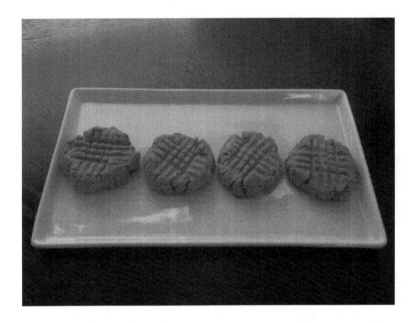

These are so good! I could eat these everyday!

1 Cup organic natural peanut butter

½ Cup Earth Balance

½ Cup maple syrup

1/3 Cup sugar

¼ Cup brown sugar

1 Teaspoon vanilla

2 Cups all purpose flour

1 Tablespoon of peanut butter powder

(Betty Louis) you can omit this if you want a less peanut buttery taste.

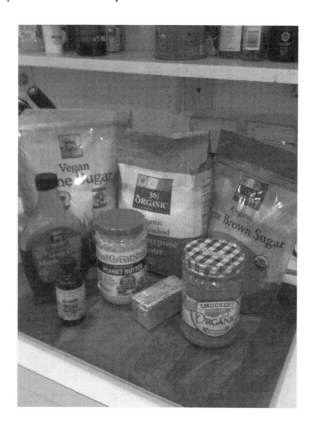

Preheat oven to 350 degrees. You can use non stick baking sheets or grease the baking sheets. Add all ingredients EXCEPT the flour and mix until fluffy and then start to add the flour. Now form the dough into small round flat circles and flatten them a bit with a fork to form a cross pattern. Bake for 15 minutes or until golden brown. Let cool for a couple minutes and then take them off the baking sheet to cool a bit more. They will be a bit dry but very tasty!

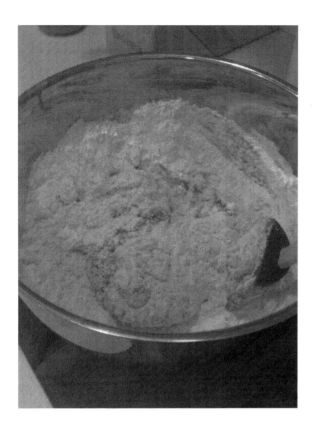

Almond Cookies

2 Cups whole wheat pastry flour

2 ½ cups ground up fine almonds

½ Teaspoon non aluminum baking powder

1 Teaspoon baking soda

2 Teaspoon almond extract

¾ Cup safflower oil

Heat oven to 350. Combine all dry ingredients in a separate bowl. Next add all the liquid ingredients. Now combine the ingredients and mix well. Roll the dough into small balls and flatten a bit on a cookie sheet and bake for 10-12 minutes or until golden brown.

Everything Bars

1/3 Cup Extra firm tofu (drained)

1/3 Cup vanilla almond milk

1/3 Cup raw sugar

1 Teaspoon vanilla extract

1 Tablespoon arrowroot powder

¼ Earth Balance

1 Cup almond meal (Finely ground almonds or graham cracker crumbs)

½ Cup pecans

½ Cup shredded coconut

½ Cup vegan white chocolate chips

½ Cup semi sweet chocolate chips

Heat oven to 350 degrees. Grease a 9 x 10 baking pan. Next melt the Earth Balance and then mix in with the almond meal or graham cracker crumbs to make a crust. Press the crust into the pan. In a vita mixer take the tofu, almond milk, sugar, arrowroot, vanilla and blend until smooth and pour on top of the crust. Next add the chocolate chips, white chocolate chips, pecans and coconut and bake for at 350 degrees for 30 minutes or until golden brown.

Pies & Puddings

Chocolate Cream Pie

Vegan Whip

Almond Butter Cream Pie

Pea Nutty Peanut Butter Pie

Blackberry Pie

Cheesecake

Chocolate Pudding

Butterscotch Pudding

Butterscotch Topping

Chocolate Cream Pie

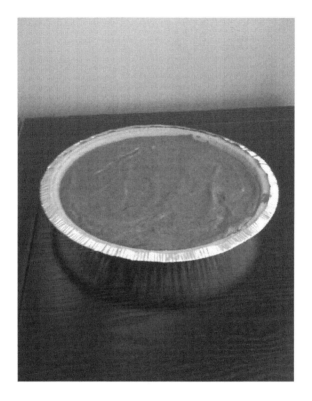

This is so easy!

1 package of silken tofu (drained as much as possible; the silken tofu is mostly drained but if you purchase other named brand it may be different)

1 ½ cup semi vegan chips or chocolate

2 Tablespoons of organic cane sugar

½ teaspoon of vanilla extract

1 vegan graham pie crust

First take the silken tofu and blend until smooth in a blender and then melt the chocolate and fold into the tofu mixture until smooth. Now pour into a premade graham crust and refrigerate until cold. Serve with vegan whip if you like.

Vegan Whip

1 Package of silken tofu

2 Tablespoons of maple syrup

2 Tablespoons of Frangelica liquor

2 Tablespoons of lemon juice

1 Teaspoon of vanilla extract

1-2 Tablespoons of almond milk

Mix all ingredients in a food processor until smooth and creamy. You may have to adjust the amount of almond milk depending on the texture of the whip cream.

Almond Butter Cream Pie

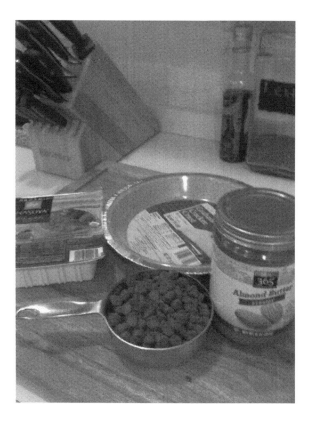

This is basically the same as the above mixture just adding almond butter.

1 Package of silken tofu

1 cup vegan chips or chocolate

½ cup Almond butter

1 Tablespoon of organic cane sugar

½ Teaspoon of vanilla extract

1 vegan graham pie crust

Take the tofu and blend until smooth and melt the chocolate and then mix in the almond butter until smooth and creamy and pour into a premade vegan pie shell of your choice!

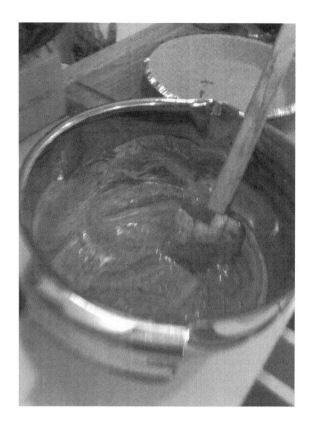

Pea Nutty Peanut Butter Pie

1 Package of silken soft tofu

3 Tablespoons of powdered peanut butter (this is great! It's from Betty Louis online)

1 Tablespoon of organic cane sugar

1 Cup melted vegan peanut butter chips

Melt the peanut butter chips in the microwave slowly or on the stove top slowly and keep stirring constantly. Mix all the rest of the ingredients in a blender until smooth and fold the melted peanut butter chips in and pour into a premade graham crust.

Blackberry Pie

Crust:

½ Cup whole wheat flour

½ Cup white unbleached flour

5 Tablespoons of water

2 Tablespoons of safflower oil

2 Tablespoons of sugar

Mix all ingredients together, cover, and set in the refrigerator while you make the filling.

Filling:

4 Cups fresh blackberries

2 Tablespoons of arrowroot

1/2 Cup of maple syrup

Mix above berry mixture

Now roll out the dough and form it to a pie pan. If you have some dough left save it to make strips for the top of the pie. Make sure to poke a few fork holes into the shell before you put the berry mixture into the pie pan. Now take the berry mixture and pour into the pie shell and put the strips on top and bake at 350 degrees for 40-45 minutes. If the top starts to get to brown make sure to cover with a piece of foil and finish baking.

*Now remember you can make the same pie with raspberries, blueberries, or your favorite berries!

Cheesecake

1 Vegan graham cracker crust

1 ½ Cup Firm Silken Tofu

1 Cup soy cream cheese

1 Cup sugar

1 Tablespoon of lemon juice

1 teaspoon of vanilla extract

½ Cup coconut milk

3 Tablespoons of arrowroot

Mix the arrowroot and coconut milk together in a small saucepan and heat until thickened. (If the mixture looks to runny make sure to add a bit more arrowroot).

Once this is done add the rest of the ingredients in a vita mixer and blend until smooth and then add the arrowroot and coconut mixture and blend again. Now pour into the pie crust and garnish with your favorite topping like cherry, raspberries, blueberries, drizzled semi sweet chocolate and refrigerate for 10 hours before serving.

*Another great idea is to freeze the pie for later!

Chocolate Pudding

1 Package of firm tofu

1 Pitted date

½ Cup organic powdered sugar

3 Tablespoons of chocolate almond milk

5 Tablespoons of cocoa powder

1 Teaspoon of vanilla extract

Blend all ingredients in a vita mixer until smooth and pour into small containers and refrigerate for 1-2 hours.

Butterscotch Pudding

1 Package of firm tofu

2 pitted dates

3 Tablespoons of almond milk

1 Teaspoon of butterscotch extract

½ cup butterscotch ice cream topping (make sure its vegan)

(Here is a recipe for butterscotch sauce if you can't find it in the store).

Butterscotch Topping

¾ Cup brown sugar

3 Tablespoons of almond milk

3 Tablespoons of brown rice syrup

¼ Cup Earth Balance

1 Teaspoon of arrowroot

Heat all ingredients in a sauce pan and keep stirring until it starts to bubble and gets to 250 degrees. Once this is done take it off the stove and allow to cool a bit before adding it to the pudding. You can also use this sauce to drizzle on your ice cream! Yum!

Now back to the real thing here the pudding. In a vita mixer add all ingredients for the pudding and blend until smooth. Transfer the mixture to small pudding containers and refrigerate for a couple hours and serve!

Frozen Treats

Frozen Chocolate Nib Bananas

Chocolate Coconut Ice Cream

Strawberry Ice Cream

Lavender & White Chocolate Ice Cream

Peanut Butter Cookies Dough Ice Cream

Chocolate Chunk Ice Cream

Banilla Bean Ice Cream

Vanilla Bean Ice Cream

Walnut, Chocolate, & Banana Ice Cream

Coffee Buzz Ice Cream

Banilla Shake

Chocolate Malt

Coffee Shake

Peanut Butter & Chocolate Shake

Frozen Chocolate Nib Bananas

3 Bananas

1 Cup Cocoa Nibs

1-1 ½ Cups of melted semi sweet chocolate

6 Wooden sticks

There is some preparation first. Take the bananas and peel them and cut them in half, put the stick in the banana so that you will have something to hold the banana with. Then dip them in the melted chocolate and roll in the cocoa nibs and freeze overnight!

Chocolate Coconut Ice Cream

1 Cup soaked cashews

1 Cup of water

½ Cup cocoa powder

2/3 Cup of agave nectar

½ teaspoon of vanilla

1 Cup soy milk

Pinch of salt

1 Frozen banana

½ Cup raw shredded coconut

Make sure to have your ice cream maker bowl frozen first (it takes about a day). Then take all of the ingredients except the coconut and mix together until smooth (in a blender or a vita mixer). Now take the mixer and add the coconut and put into the freezer bowl and mix until done. Then take out of the freezer bowl and serve now or put in another container and freeze for later! This tastes just like ice cream!

Strawberry Ice Cream

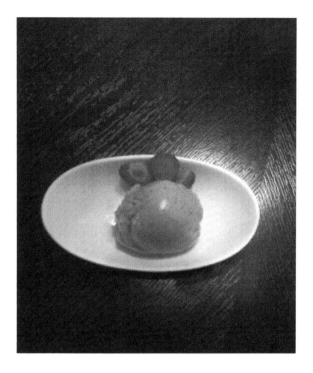

1 Quart of strawberries (with tops off)

1 Can coconut milk (if you want a lower fat version you can use half coconut milk and half almond milk)

½ Plus 1/8 Cup of organic sugar (depends on how ripe the strawberries)

2   Teaspoons of vanilla extract

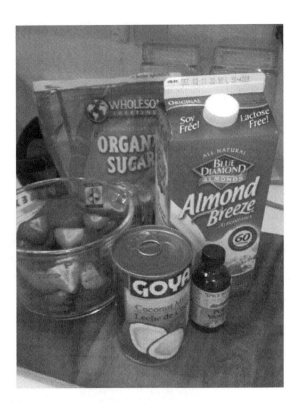

Mix all ingredients in a vita mixer until smooth. Then cool in the refrigerator for 2 hours and then use your ice cream mixer to make awesome ice cream.

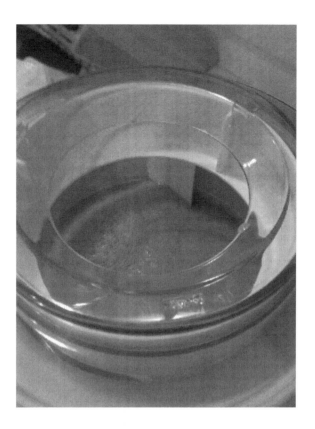

*For blackberry or any other berry ice cream use the same ingredients except swap the strawberries for the strawberries.

This recipe is more like a sorbet and does melt fast right out of the ice cream maker so you may want to freeze it for a couple hours before serving.

Lavender & White Chocolate Ice Cream

1 ¼ Cup vanilla soymilk

¼ Cup fresh lavender flowers

1 Can coconut milk

½ Cup sugar

1 Cup vegan white chocolate chips

I love white chocolate and lavender in latte's, hot chocolate, and now in my ice cream!

Heat the soymilk in a small pan along with the lavender on low heat until it begins to boil and then let sit for 15-20 minutes. Strain the lavender from this mixture and set back on the stove on low heat and gradually add the white chocolate chips. Add the rest of the ingredients and place in the refrigerator for several hours and then add to the ice cream maker. Serve right away or place in a freezer container and have some later!

Peanut Butter Cookie Dough Ice Cream

This is one of my favorites! Make the dough from the peanut butter cookies that I have in this book first and roll them into small little balls and save for later. (About 1 Cup; you can bake the rest of the dough into cookies for a garnish or just make half of the recipe).

1 Can of coconut milk

1 Cup hemp milk

½ Cup sugar

½ Cup peanut butter

Mix all ingredients except the cookie dough in a bowl and refrigerate for 3 hours. When that is done take the mixture out of the refrigerator and use the ice cream maker to make the ice cream. When the mixture is done add the small pieces of cookie dough and freeze for a couple hours and serve!

Chocolate Chunk Ice Cream

1 Cup soaked Brazil nuts (for 1-2 hours)

1 Cup of water

½ Cup cocoa powder

1 Cups almond milk

2/3 Cup of agave nectar

½ teaspoon of vanilla

Pinch of salt

1 Frozen banana

½ Cup semi sweet chocolate chopped into small pieces

First take all of the ingredients except the chopped chocolate and mix in a vita mixer. Then add to your frozen ice cream bowl and mix until it looks like ice cream. After that take out of the bowl and add the pieces of chocolate and serve. This will be really creamy and tasty!

Banilla Bean Ice Cream

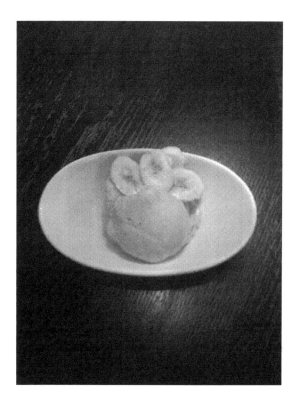

1 Cup soaked raw cashews (for 1-2 hours)

1 Cup of water

1 Cup almond milk

2/3 Cup of agave nectar

½ teaspoon of vanilla

½ of a Vanilla bean

Pinch of salt

1 Frozen banana

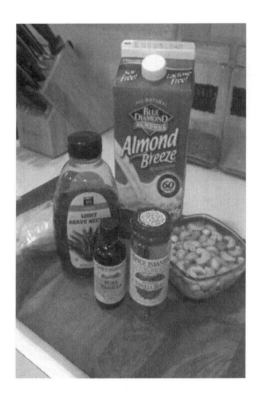

First take the vanilla bean and scrap the inside of the bean and add that to the rest of the ingredients and mix in a vita mixer. Then add that mixture to the ice cream maker and serve when done or freeze for later!

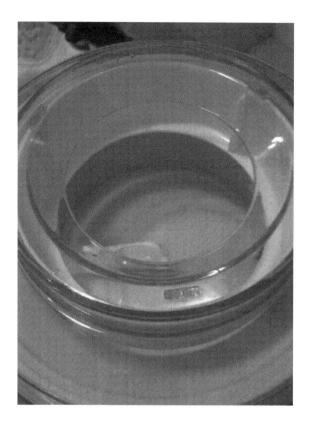

Vanilla Bean Ice Cream

1 Cup soaked raw cashews

2/3 Cup agave nectar

Pinch of salt

1 Cup vanilla almond milk

1 Teaspoon of vanilla

½ Vanilla bean

Mix all ingredients in a vita mixer and then refrigerate for a couple hours. After the mixture has cooled for a couple of hours take it out of the refrigerator and mix as you would in your ice cream maker. Either serve right away or freeze in another container for later.

Walnut, Chocolate, & Banana Ice Cream

1 Cup soaked raw walnuts (for 1-2 hours)

1 Cup of water

1 Cup almond milk

2/3 Cup of agave nectar

½ teaspoon of vanilla extract

Pinch of salt

1 Frozen banana

½ Cup chopped chocolate chunks

Take all ingredients except the chocolate chunks and mix in a vita mixer. Then use your ice cream maker to make smooth ice cream. When it is done add the chopped chocolate and freeze in another container or serve!

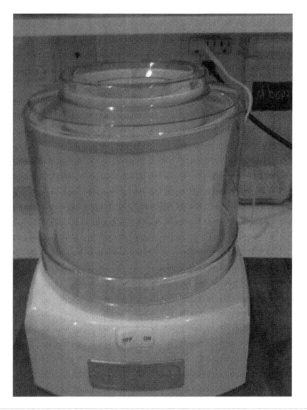

Coffee Buzz Ice Cream

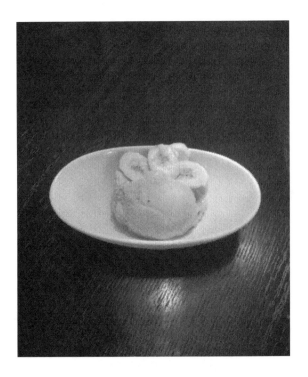

1 Cup of raw Brazil nuts soaked for 2-3 hours and then drained

1 ½ Cup of coffee with vanilla soy creamer

½ Cup of hemp milk

½ Cup agave nectar

Pinch of salt

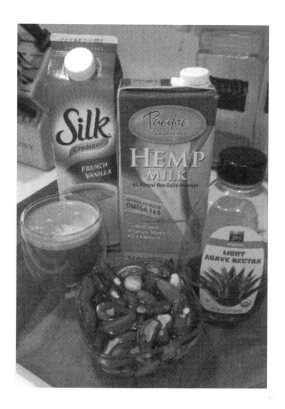

Mix all ingredients in a vita mixer and the cool in the refrigerator for a couple hours and then mix in your ice cream maker. Serve!

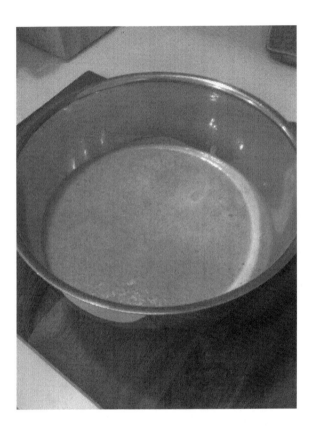

Banilla Shake

2 Scoops of the Banilla Ice Cream

½ Cup vanilla almond milk

Mix the ingredients up in a vita mixer and serve! Yummy!

Chocolate Malt

3   Scoops of Chocolate Chunk Ice Cream

½ Cup chocolate almond milk

1 Scoop of malt flavoring

Mix all ingredients up in a vita mixer and serve!

Coffee Shake

2 Scoops of Coffee Buzz Ice Cream

½ Cup vanilla almond milk

½ Cup of coffee

Mix all ingredients in a vita mixer and serve!

Peanut Butter & Chocolate Shake

1 Scoop Peanut Butter Cookie Dough Ice Cream

1 Scoop of Chocolate Chunk Ice Cream

¾ Cup vanilla almond milk

2 Tablespoons of peanut butter

Mix all ingredients together with a vita mixer and serve!

Sweet Drinks

Pumpkin Pie Smoothie

Mojito Punch

Pineapple Mint Smoothie

Chocolate Blackberry Surprise

Coffee Cooler

Chocolate Banana Dream

Peanut Butter Splash

Banana Crème Latte

Pumpkin Pie Smoothie

1 Package of silken soft tofu

1 Can of organic pumpkin puree

1 teaspoon of cinnamon

1 Cup of ice

1/8-1/4 Cup organic orange juice

Mix all ingredients in a blender and drink up!

This makes two large glasses or four small ones. If you want more protein you can add a vanilla vegan powder mix like Sun Warrior Vegan Meal or your favorite vegan vanilla protein mix.

Mojito Punch

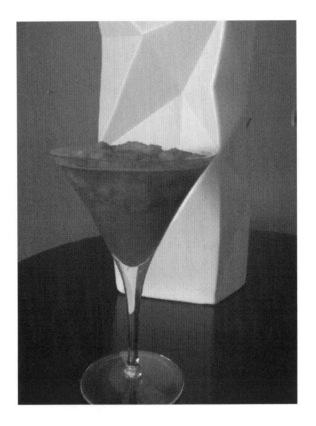

1/8-1/4 Cup Mint Leaves

3 Tablespoons of maple sugar

1 Cup of ice

½ Cup of Lime Juice (more if you like it tart)

Mix all ingredients to in a vita mixer or blender and serve with a mint sprig!

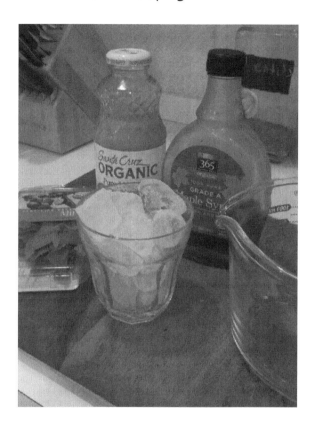

Pineapple Mint Smoothie

1 Cup of fresh pineapple

1/8 Cup of mint

1 Cup of ice

1 Cup of almond, hemp or hazelnut milk

½ Frozen banana

A splash of orange juice

Mix all ingredients in a vita mixer or blender and serve with a slice of pineapple!

Chocolate Blackberry Surprise

1 Cup chocolate hemp milk

1 Cup Frozen blackberries

¼ Cup of orange juice

1 Cup of ice

¼ Cup cocoa nibs

Mix all ingredients in a vita mixer or blender and serve!

Coffee Cooler

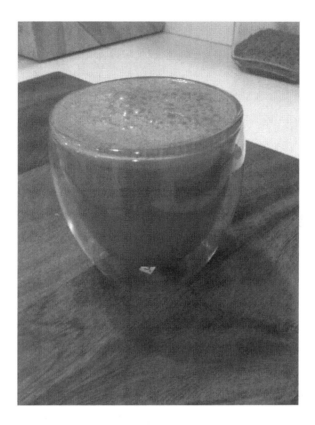

1 Cup cold coffee or if you like it stronger a couple of shots of espresso works really good

1 Cup ice

1 Cup chocolate almond milk (or a just add a scoop of cacao powder to regular almond milk; it will be less sweeter this way)

Another thing that is good is to change out the almond milk for vanilla soy creamer especially if you like a sweeter drink.

Mix all ingredients together and serve.

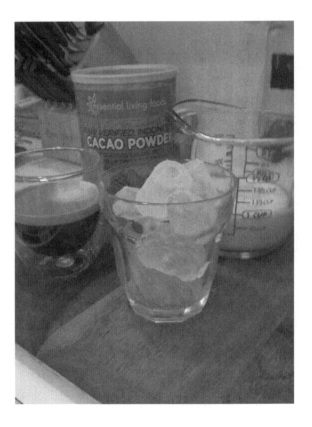

Chocolate Banana Dream

1 Frozen banana

1 Cup chocolate hemp milk

1 Tablespoon of almond butter

1 Cup of ice

1 Tablespoon of hemp oil

Mix all ingredients together and serve!

Peanut Butter Splash

½ Cup peanut butter

1 Cup ice

1 Cup vanilla almond milk

½ Frozen banana

Splash of orange juice

Mix all ingredients together in a vita mixer or a blender.

Banana Crème Latte

1 Double Espresso

1 Scoop of Banana Vanilla Ice Cream

Make your espresso. Then add a scoop of the ice cream and wait a minute for it to melt and sip on a delicious drink!

Some Helpful Websites

www.veganmainstream.com Great for vegan businesses! I was interviewed on this site!

www.vegan.com

www.supervegan.com

www.goveg.com

www.kidbean.com (vegan kid clothing and accessories)

www.vegancoach.com

www.vegansociety.com

www.findaspring.com

www.cosmeticdatabase.com

www.etsy.com This site has particular sellers that have etsyveg next to their items if they support the vegan lifestyle or their products are vegan!

www.vegnews.com This is a great website to help promote your vegan business along with great tips on a vegan diet!

www.veganstore.com They have great vegan white chocolate chips!

www.veganoutreach.org

Some Helpful Phone Apps

Vegan Yum Yum. This app lets you search, view, and organize all your favorite vegan recipes.

VeganXpress. If you are on the go a lot then this app will work for you. Veganxpress lets you see what restaurants and fast food places have vegan fare.

VegScan. This is a great app that you can scan the barcode to check to see if the food product is vegan or vegetarian! So cool!

HappyCow. This is one of my favorites! I love the website and the app! This app lets you have vegan and vegetarian restaurants on the go. There is an interactive map that shows you where the restaurants and stores are located. There is also phone numbers, directions, and their websites. You can also share on facebook & twitter! I big bonus if you find something really great!

WholeFoodsMarket. This is a great app that allows you to search for recipes, with nutritional information, add ingredients to your shopping list, store locator! This is great if you are traveling!

Eden Recipes. This is great for recipes and sharing them on facebook!

Gardein Recipes. I love these things! They are so tasty! This is a great app if you just don't know what goes with a gardein.

Cruelty-Free. This is a great app for shopping animal free!

VegWeb. This app has vegan recipes.

Veggie Passport. This is a great app if you are traveling and you want to explain what you can or cannot eat. You can choose your language (there are lots to choose from) and then chose the message you want to tell the waiter. This is very useful and weighs less than a phrase book.

There are so many apps out there! Plus they change daily! Just keep up to date! It's the greatest way to keep your diet in check!

VEGAN COOKINGS CLASSES AND SCHOOLS

CALIFORNIA

Spork Foods
7494 Santa Monica Blvd Ste 302
W Hollywood, CA 90046
www.sporkonline.com

Living Light Culinary Arts Institute
704 N Harrison
Fort Bragg, CA 95437
www.rawfoodchef.com

Bay Area Vegetarians
PO Box 700
Vallejo, CA 94590-0069
www.bayareaveg.org

The New School of Cooking
8690 Washington Blvd
Culver City, CA 90232
310-842-9702
www.newschoolofcooking.com

Hip Cooks
642 Moulton Ave
Los Angeles, CA 90031
323-222-3663
www.hipcooks.com
They are also located in Portland, OR, Seattle, WA, East and West LA.

HAWAAII

Vegan Fusion
www.veganfusion.com
PO Box 1119
Kapaa, HI 96746

NEW YORK

Natural Gourmet Institute for Health & Culinary Arts
48 W 21st St 2nd Floor
New York, NY 10010
212-645-5170
www.naturalgourmetinstitute.com

NORTH CAROLINA

Lenoresnatural.com
Lenore Baum
164 Ox Creek Rd

Weaverville, NC 28787
828-645-1412

VIRGINIA

Mimi Clarks Vegan Cooking Classes
9302 Hallston Ct
Fairfax Station, VA 22039
703-643-2713
www.veggourmet.wordpress.com

TEXAS

The Natural Epicurean Academy of Culinary Arts
1700 S Lamar Blvd
Austin, TX 78704
512-476-2276
www.naturalepicurean.com

CANADA

Live Nutrition Cooking School
5 Kitsilano Crescent
Richmond Hill
Ontario, L4C 5A4
905-884-9112
www.livenutritionschool.com

The Vegan Vegetarian Cooking School

3988 Galloway Frt Rd
Elko, BC V0B 1 J0
250-529-7750

ENGLAND

Cordon Vert Vegetarian Cookery School
Parkdale
Dunham Rd
Altrinchaum
Cheshire, England
01619252014
www.cordonvert.co.uk
(They are a vegetarian school but they make exceptions for vegan)

About the Author

B.S. in Physical Anthropology, Minor in Business, and Art Institute of Fort Lauderdale Culinary Arts Degree.

Advocate for organic, vegetarian, vegan, and raw food diets. I have been a vegetarian/vegan/raw foodist for over 20 years. Owner of Sunny Cabana Publishing, L.L.C. and a published author of living foods and raw food recipe books for Recipes 4 Raw Food, The Vivacious Vegan, & The Vivacious Vegan Desserts.

Have several websites to help people who are interested in healthy eating www.Recipes4RawFood.com, and www.RawFoodForToday.com.

Owner of www.RawFoodsAssociation.com and www.SunnyCabanaPublishing.com

Follow me on Facebook: facebook.com/sunnycabanapublishing

Email: SunnyCabanaPublishing@gmail.com

Or TheVivaciousVegan@gmail.com

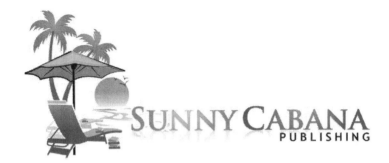

Index

A
Agave Nectar Page 22, 47, 87, 94, 95, 97, 98, 100
Almonds Page 34, 63, 67, 69
Apples Page 23, 33, 36, 37, 38, 40, 41, 42
Arrowroot Page 22, 53, 68, 69, 79, 81, 82

B

Bananas Page 23, 25, 31, 32, 85, 87, 89, 94, 97, 98, 99, 105, 110, 113, 114
Blueberries Page 39, 40, 79, 81
Brazil Nuts Page 94, 100
Bread Page 5, 25, 31, 45, 47
Brittle Page 49, 63
Brown Rice Syrup Page 17, 63
Butterscotch Page 71, 82

C
Cakes Page 5, 7, 16, 20, 25, 27, 29, 33, 34, 35, 37, 43, 44, 45, 71, 80
Cacao powder Page 111
Carrots Page 36
Cashews Page 87, 95, 97
Cheesecake Page 71, 80
Chocolate Page 22, 25, 27, 28, 30, 41, 42, 45, 49, 54, 55, 56, 63, 69, 71, 73, 74, 77, 81, 85, 87, 92, 94, 98, 99, 103, 104, 110, 111, 113
Coconut Page 22, 25, 33, 34, 69, 80, 85, 87, 88, 89, 92, 93
Coffee Page 25, 27, 29, 85, 100, 103, 105, 111
Cookies Page 5, 45, 49, 59, 60, 61, 64, 67, 68, 85, 93, 104
Cupcakes Page 25, 43

D
Dates Page 16, 22, 36, 58, 82

E

F

Flaxseeds Page 23
Flour Page 5, 19, 20, 22, 28, 31, 33, 34, 35, 36, 39, 40, 42, 43, 44, 46, 51, 52, 53, 55, 57, 61, 65, 66, 67, 78
Food Processor Page 16, 22, 74
Frosting Page 25, 37, 44, 45

G

H

Hazelnuts Page 36, 37, 39, 40, 42, 54, 61, 110
Hemp Page 28, 36, 93, 100

I

Ice Cream Maker Page 22, 88, 91, 92, 93, 97, 98, 99, 101
Ice Cream Page 7, 23, 82, 85, 87, 88, 89, 90, 91, 92, 93, 94, 95, 97-104, 114

J

L
Lavender Page 85, 92
Lemon Page 49, 51, 52, 74, 80

M
Maple Syrup Page 16, 17, 22, 28, 29, 31, 36, 37, 46, 58, 64, 74, 79, 108
Mint Page 45, 105, 108, 109
Muffins Page 5, 21, 25, 38, 40, 41, 42, 43, 44

N

O

Oats Page 22, 49, 57, 60, 61
Orange Page 14, 25, 34, 35, 107, 110, 113

P
Peanut Page 49, 55, 63, 64, 65, 71, 77, 78, 85, 93, 104, 113
Pecans Page 25, 29, 31, 38, 39, 40, 60, 61, 69
Pineapple Page 25, 27, 29, 30, 105, 109, 110
Pudding Page 5, 71, 81, 82, 83
Pumpkin Page 105, 107

Q

R

Raisins Page 36, 58, 61
Raspberries Page 42, 79, 81

S
Strawberry Page 85, 89
Sugar Page 5, 15-17, 19, 23, 33-37, 39-44, 51-55, 60-64, 68, 69, 74, 76, 77, 78, 80, 81, 82, 89, 92

T
Tofu Page 7, 13, 14, 22, 52, 6, 69, 73, 74-77, 80-82, 107

U

V
Vanilla Page 25, 28, 34-37, 39, 40, 42, 43, 44, 54, 55, 58, 61, 65, 68, 69, 74, 76, 80, 81, 85, 88, 89, 92, 94, 95, 96, 97, 98, 100, 103, 104, 107, 112, 113
Vegan Whip Page 74

W

Walnut Page 37, 54, 55, 58, 85, 98

Y

Z

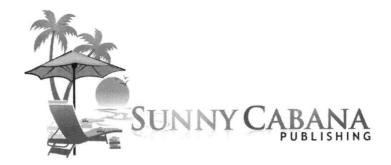

The Vivacious Vegan

$13.95

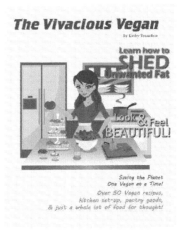

Awesome Raw Food Guide

$15.95

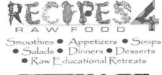

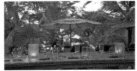

80 Awesome Raw Food Recipes You Can't Live Without

$14.95

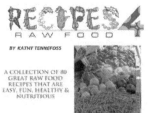

Check out more of Sunny Cabana Publishing books at www.SunnyCabanaPublishing.com

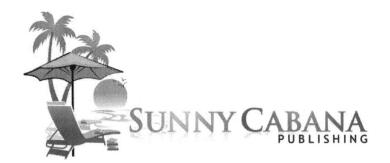

Made in the USA
Charleston, SC
11 December 2011